SLIMFAST DIE'
BOOK

Your Comprehensive Guide To Healthy Weight Management And Lifestyle Changes, SlimFast

TIMOTHY ANDERSON

Contents

CHAPTER ONE

An Introductory

Meal replacement shakes, snacks, and bars are all part of the SlimFast line of weight loss products.

By substituting SlimFast products for two meals per day and eating one healthy meal and three low-calorie snacks, the SlimFast diet can aid in weight loss.

SlimFast products are high in protein and fiber but low in calories, allowing dieters to feel full on a smaller calorie intake. The shakes are versatile, as they can be made with either milk or water, and the snacks and bars are made to be eaten on the move.

Through its website and social media channels, SlimFast provides not just products, but also assistance and guidance in the form of recipes, meal plans, and weight loss ideas.

It is recommended that before beginning any weight loss program, you speak with a medical practitioner and keep in mind that SlimFast and other weight loss products should be taken in conjunction with a healthy diet and lifestyle.

What Makes Slimfast Tick?

In order for the SlimFast plan to be effective, you must consume fewer calories than your body needs on a daily basis for weight maintenance (a "calorie deficit").

Putting the body into a caloric deficit causes it to use fat reserves for fuel, which might result in gradual weight reduction.

Replacement of two daily meals with SlimFast products, which are typically fewer in calories than a standard meal, creates a calorie deficit in the SlimFast program.

A SlimFast shake, on the other hand, may only have 200–300 calories, while a standard meal may have 500–700 calories. You can drastically cut your daily calorie consumption by using SlimFast products to replace two meals.

Meal replacements are just one part of the SlimFast plan; participants are also encouraged to consume one healthy meal and three low-calorie snacks daily.

In this way, you can acquire the nutrients you need while also maintaining a caloric deficit that aids in weight loss.

SlimFast is formulated to be high in protein and fiber, two nutrients that contribute to satiety and a decrease in harmful food cravings.

The program also stresses the importance of exercise and encourages participants to maintain an active lifestyle.

The SlimFast regimen can help you lose weight, but it is not a silver bullet and should not be used in isolation from a good diet and exercise routine. Before beginning any weight loss program, it is recommended that you consult a healthcare expert.

CHAPTER TWO

Advantages

If you are looking to slim down and boost your health, the SlimFast diet may be the way to go. Possible SlimFast diet advantages are as follows:

• The SlimFast program's ease is a major selling point. Meal replacement shakes, snacks, and bars may be quickly grabbed on the move, making them a viable option for people who are too busy to cook nutritious meals.

• SlimFast is a wonderful alternative for people who have trouble sticking to regular diets because it is easy to follow and involves nothing in the way of preparation.

• SlimFast's portion-controlled meals and snacks can teach dieters to eat less by providing them with a framework for doing so.

• SlimFast's systematic approach to weight loss is designed to keep dieters on track and ultimately successful.

5. Protein and fiber content is often high in SlimFast products, making consumers feel full longer and maybe reducing their desire for harmful snacks.

• A network of people with similar weight loss goals is available to you as part of the SlimFast program. Those participating in the program may find this an additional source of inspiration and responsibility.

The SlimFast regimen is not for everyone, and it is best when it is used in conjunction with other healthy habits like exercise and a well-balanced diet. Before beginning any weight loss program, it is recommended that you consult a healthcare expert.

Shakes And Bars That Substitute Meals

The SlimFast plan relies heavily on meal replacement shakes and snacks. These items are intended to be consumed in place of two meals per day and often have fewer calories than a full meal.

SlimFast shakes are available in a wide range of tastes and may be prepared with either milk or water.

Due to their high protein and fiber content, they may aid with satiety. Vitamins and minerals have been included to the shakes to assist with nutritional upkeep.

SlimFast bars are another option for replacing meals on the fly because of their portability and nutritional density.

The bars, like the shakes, are packed with protein and fiber to keep you feeling full and content between meals.

The portion control in both the shakes and the bars can aid in the process of learning to eat less at each meal.

A healthcare practitioner should be consulted before beginning any weight loss program, and meal replacement products should not be utilized as the primary source of nutrition.

CHAPTER THREE
Meals And Snacks Available

In addition to the two meal replacement shakes or bars per day, participants in the SlimFast program are encouraged to eat one healthy meal and three low-calorie snacks each day.

Some meal and snack ideas that work with the SlimFast plan are listed below.

Food choices:

• Fruit that is just been picked (apples, pears, bananas, berries, etc.).

• Raw veggies (such as celery, bell peppers, and carrot sticks).

• Yogurt or cottage cheese that is low in fat.

• Toasted brie.

• Puffed rice,

• Popcorn popped in the air.

• Eggs that have been cooked to a hard state.

Menu Selections:

• Chicken, fish, and veggies cooked on the grill.

• A healthy stir-fry with lean protein and greens.

• Vegetable-packed salad topped with a lean protein source (chicken, turkey, shrimp, etc.).

• A broth including lean meat and greens.

• Salad or boiled vegetables and a turkey or vegetarian burger.

• Vegetable omelets or frittatas with low-fat cheese.

When following the SlimFast diet, it is important to focus on eating lean protein, lots of veggies, and moderate amounts of nutritious carbohydrates. Be mindful of serving sizes and try to limit your daily calorie intake.

Meal-Planning Examples

Two daily SlimFast menus are shown below as examples.

Menu Option 1:

Breakfast:

• (From 200-300 calories) SlimFast shake.

Snack:

• Sliced apples with peanut butter (150 calories).

Lunch:

• Veggie roast with grilled chicken breast (300 calories).

Snack:

• A SlimFast bar (between 100 and 150 calories).

Dinner:

• Salmon and quinoa bake (400 calories) with steamed greens.

Snack:

• 50 calorie little cup of mixed berries.

Calorie intake: between 1200 and 1300 daily.

Menu Option 2:

Breakfast:

• (From 200-300 calories) SlimFast shake.

Snack:

• 1.150-calorie serving of hummus and carrot sticks.

Lunch:

• Salad with turkey burger (350 calories).

Snack:

• A SlimFast bar (between 100 and 150 calories).

Dinner:

• Brown-rice and vegetable stir-fry (400 calories) with lean protein (chicken or tofu).

Snack:

• One hundred calorie serving of low-fat Greek yogurt and fresh fruit.

Calorie intake: between 1200 and 1300 daily

Keep in mind that these menus are merely examples and can be modified to suit your specific requirements and tastes.

To maintain your health and well-being, it is crucial that you pay attention to your body's needs and provide it with the nutrition and energy it requires.

Slimfast As Part Of A Healthy Routine

Although SlimFast was created with weight loss in mind, it can also be used to support long-term health and wellness. Here are some suggestions for making SlimFast a permanent part of your healthy routine:

• Get moving: Physical activity improves health in many ways, including helping people keep off the weight they have lost. Make an effort to get at least 30 minutes of exercise every day, whether it is walking, jogging, cycling, or something else.

• The convenience of SlimFast products should not detract from the need of a diet rich in lean protein, whole grains, fruits, and vegetables. Nutrient-dense and filling, these foods are a great choice.

• Even if you are not following the SlimFast plan to a T, it is still crucial to watch your portion sizes to keep from gaining weight.

To achieve nutritional balance, try to estimate portion amounts using measuring cups, a food scale, or even just your hand.

• Drinking adequate water is crucial to your health and might make you feel more satiated and give you more energy. Try to drink 8 glasses of water daily and cut out on sugary drinks in favor of water or low-calorie drinks.

• It is crucial to be patient with yourself and to set reasonable expectations, as both weight loss and good living require time. Acknowledge your achievements and keep working toward permanent improvements.

Keep in mind that SlimFast is but one method among many that can help you lead a healthier life. It is crucial to tune in to your physical requirements and make decisions accordingly.

CHAPTER FOUR

Slimfast Food And Drink
Macronutrient Breakdown

SlimFast products have a wide range of macronutrient breakdowns due to the wide variety of brands and flavors available. In general, SlimFast products have the following macronutrient breakdown.

1. Replace-Your-Meal Shakes:

• 180-200 kcal/serving.

• 10-20 grams of protein.

• 18-25 grams of carbohydrates.

• 4-5 grams of fiber.

• 5-9 grams of fat.

2. Bars that Can Replace Meals:

• Energy level: 190-220.

• 8-10 grams of protein.

Energy: 19-26 g Carbohydrates.

• Fiber, 7 to 13 grams.

• The Fat Content Is Between 6 and 9 Grams.

SlimFast products are created to have less calories and fewer carbohydrates than a regular meal.

A calorie deficit is essential for weight loss, and this may help you get there. However, in order to maintain optimal health, it is necessary to ensure that you are consuming a sufficient quantity of nutritious whole foods.

If you have any preexisting health ailments or concerns, it is highly recommended that you speak with a doctor before beginning any weight loss program.

Measured Against Suggested Daily Allowances

A person's recommended daily intake of macronutrients (protein, carbs, and fat) changes with age, sex, height, weight, and level of physical activity, among other things.

However, if you stick to a diet of 2,000 calories per day, here are some general recommendations for appropriate intakes:

• 50–175 grams of protein (10–35 percent of total calories).

• 225–325 grams of carbohydrates (45–65 percent of total calories).

• 44-77 grams of fat (20-35% of total calories).

SlimFast foods are moderate in protein and fat, and include less calories and fewer carbohydrates than recommended. If you are trying to lose weight, this may help you achieve the calorie deficit you need.

However, in order to maintain optimal health, it is necessary to ensure that you are consuming a sufficient quantity of nutritious whole foods.

SlimFast dieters should consult a doctor to determine whether or not they are getting enough of certain nutrients while on the diet.

Effects That Could Go Wrong

Although the SlimFast program has been shown to be safe for the vast majority of users, it is possible for some people to feel discomfort. Some potential adverse effects include:

• Some people may experience hunger or cravings while on the SlimFast regimen, despite the fact that the products are made to be satisfying.

• Deficiencies in essential nutrients: Because SlimFast products have less calories and carbohydrates than regular meals, it is crucial to ensure adequate consumption of healthy whole foods.

• When beginning the program, some people may have digestive difficulties such gas, bloating, or diarrhea. This could be because of the large amount of fiber in certain SlimFast products.

• Switching to SlimFast products, which contain various amounts of caffeine, may cause headaches or other symptoms of caffeine withdrawal in persons who normally consume large amounts of caffeine.

• Some people may have adverse responses to SlimFast products because they contain allergens including milk, soy, or nuts.

If you have any preexisting health ailments or concerns, you should discuss the SlimFast program with your doctor before beginning it, as you should with any weight loss program or dietary modification.

If you have any adverse reactions while on the program, you should stop immediately and consult a doctor.

CHAPTER FIVE

When Is The Slimfast Diet Not A Good Idea?

While SlimFast is healthy for the majority of dieters, there are some groups who should either not follow the diet or make adjustments to it. For example:

• Women who are pregnant or breastfeeding have unique nutritional needs for both themselves and their infants, and the SlimFast plan may not provide enough of the right foods to meet those needs.

• For children and teenagers, the SlimFast diet may not provide enough of certain nutrients to support proper growth and development.

• People with preexisting medical conditions People with preexisting medical conditions may need to make adjustments to the SlimFast program or should not use it at all, including those with diabetes, liver or kidney disease, or eating disorders.

If you have any preexisting health ailments or concerns, you should consult a doctor before beginning the program.

• Some people may have adverse reactions to or intolerances to the substances found in SlimFast products, including as milk, soy, and nuts.

• Because of its focus on weight loss, the SlimFast program may not be suitable for people who are already underweight or who have a history of eating problems.

Before beginning any weight loss program, it is recommended that you consult a doctor, especially if you have preexisting health conditions or concerns.

Conclusion

The SlimFast diet, in a nutshell, is a weight loss plan in which you replace one or two meals per day with meal replacement shakes or bars and then eat a normal, healthy meal for the other meal(s).

The regimen is structured to supply appropriate nourishment while producing the calorie deficit essential for weight loss.

SlimFast products contain modest amounts of protein and fat and less calories and carbohydrates than the average meal.

Although this can be useful for reducing caloric intake, it is essential to ensure adequate nutritional intake from whole meals in order to maintain good health.

SlimFast is thought to be safe for most people, although it may cause hunger, nutrient deficiencies, digestive difficulties, headaches, or allergic responses in a small percentage.

If you have any preexisting health ailments or concerns, you should consult a doctor before beginning the program.

When combined with other weight loss strategies, such as a healthy diet and regular exercise, SlimFast has been shown to be effective.

THE END

Printed in Great Britain
by Amazon